Keto Diet For Women

An Essential Guide To The Keto Diet
Cookbook After 50 As A Senior
Women To Regain Metabolism And
Stay Healthy Quick And Easy.

Written By

Winifred Campbell

Table of Contents

INTRODUCTION

Thank you for purchasing this book!

Here are some tips to get started:

Consult a nutrition specialist. This book is a very valuable tool to get an idea of what a ketogenic diet is, what the benefits are, how to avoid classic mistakes. It is a complete guide, with which, if studied well, you will certainly be able to set your diet according to your daily needs. However, consulting a doctor is never a bad idea, you can discuss your opinions and can give you valuable advice. I recommend consulting your doctor especially in cases of health problems and in cases where you have never been on a diet.

Take "fats" from unrefined foods (such as olive oil, avocado, walnuts). It has already been well said but I will never tire of repeating it: the quality of food is fundamental; you cannot think of obtaining concrete results (from any diet) if you do not eat quality food. Diets are based on scientific concepts, which give incredible results if you carefully follow the principles on which it is founded. It is not the magic wand, you will not lose weight from day to day, you will have to be persevering, even if not above all, in choosing the quality of the food.

Don't forget to eat starchy vegetables.

Enjoy your reading!

Flank Steak Skillet Barbecued

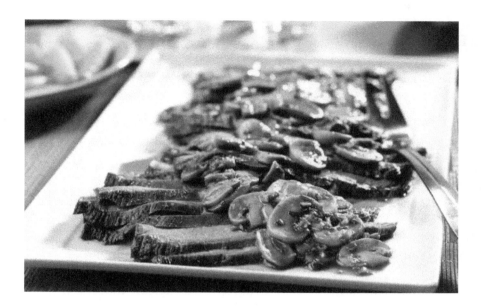

Preparation Time: 15 Minutes

Cooking Time: 10 Minutes

Servings: 4-6

Ingredients:

- Crude flank steak on butcher paper

- 1/2 pound flank steak

- Salt

- Naturally ground dark pepper

- Dry mustard

- Relaxed margarine

Direction:

1. Tenderize the steak with shallow cuts: Remove the steak from the fridge a half hour before cooking.

2. Remove any extreme connective tissue on the outside of the steak.

3. Utilizing the tip of a sharp blade, stick little cuts into the meat, practically completely through. The cuts ought to be at an edge, toward the grain of the meat as the blade tip is going in. The cuts ought to be about an inch separated from one another.

4. Turn the steak over and rehash the cuts on the opposite side. Ensure that the cuts you are making on this side are corresponding with the cuts you made on the opposite side, else you may cut over a current cut, and wind up jabbing a gap through the meat.

5. Rub with salt, pepper, dry mustard, and spread: Sprinkle one side of the steak with salt and crisply ground pepper. Sprinkle the steak with dry mustard. Rub a tablespoon of margarine everywhere throughout the side of the steak. Turn the steak over and rehash with the dry mustard, pepper, and margarine. Rub flank steak with dry mustard rub flank steak with spread

6. Sear steak in hot skillet: Heat an enormous cast iron griddle on high warmth. Spot steak in hot container. Let singe for 2 to 3 minutes until very much cooked.

7. Place flank steak in fricasseeing pan sear flank steak in griddle

8. Go through tongs to lift to check whether pleasantly caramelized. Assuming this is the case, flip to the opposite side and let burn for 2 to 3 minutes.

9. Turn flank steak over in pan sear flank steak in skillet

10. Remove from heat: Remove the skillet from the warmth and let the steak keep on cooking for 5 to 10 minutes in the lingering warmth of the container (expecting you are utilizing solid metal, if not, bring down the warmth to low).

11. Check for doneness: Use your fingertips to check for doneness or embed a meat thermometer into the thickest piece of the steak - 120°F for uncommon, 125°F for uncommon, or 130°F for medium uncommon. Flank steak ought to be served uncommon or medium uncommon, else it might be excessively dry.

12. In the event that the steak isn't done what's necessary just as you would prefer, return the steak and container to medium high warmth for a couple of moments.

13. Let the steak rest: Remove the steak from the dish to a cutting board and let rest for 10 minutes, secured with aluminum foil.

14. Thinly cut: Cut the meat in slim cuts, at an edge, over the grain of the meat. (Along these lines you get through the extreme long muscle strands.)

15. Cutting flank steak: 8 Boil juices, deglaze skillet, add margarine to make sauce: Any juices that leave the meat while cutting or resting, come back to the dish. Return the skillet to a burner on high warmth and deglaze the container with a little water, scraping up any sautéed bits. When the water has generally come down, add a little margarine to the prospect pleasant sauce.

16. Orchestrate the cut meat on a serving plate and pour the deglazed container squeezes over the meat.

Nutrition:

- **Calories:** 128 Cal

- **Fat:** 21 g

- **Carbs:** 4 g

- **Protein:** 2 g

- **Fiber:** 5 g

Avocados stuffed with Crap

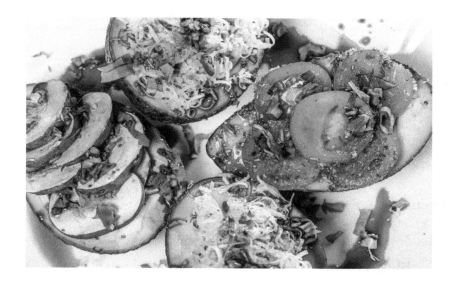

Preparation Time: 20 Minutes

Cooking Time: 50 Minutes

Servings: 4

Ingredients:

- 1 pound boneless, skinless chicken bosom

- ⅓ cup low-fat plain Greek yogurt

- ¼ cup mayonnaise

- 1 tablespoon slashed crisp tarragon or 1 teaspoon dried

- ¾ teaspoon salt

- ½ teaspoon ground pepper

- 1 cup diced celery

- 1 cup seedless red grapes, divided (discretionary)

- ¼ cup toasted slashed walnuts

- 2 firm ready avocados, divided and pitted

Direction:

1. Spot chicken in an enormous pan and add enough water to cover. Bring to a stew over medium warmth. Diminish warmth to keep up a stew, spread and cook until the chicken registers 165 degrees F with a moment read thermometer, 12 to 15 minutes. Move to a cutting board. Let remain until sufficiently cool to deal with, at that point hack or shred. Refrigerate until chilly, around 30 minutes.

2. To serve, fill every avocado half with around 1/2 cup chicken plate of mixed greens. (Refrigerate the additional chicken plate of mixed greens for as long as 3 days.)

Nutrition:

- **Calories:** 308 Cal
- **Fat:** 22 g
- **Carbs:** 6 g
- **Protein:** 8 g
- **Fiber:** 4 g

Blackened Chicken Salad

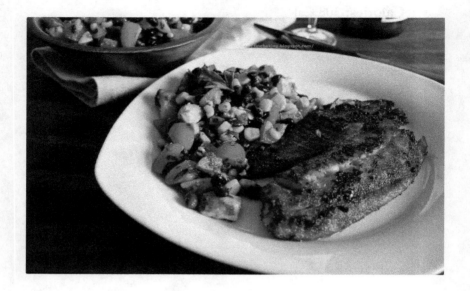

Preparation Time: 5 Minutes

Cooking Time: Minutes

Servings: 4

Ingredients:

- 2 cups cooked chicken bosom, slashed

- 4 tbsp. nonfat plain yogurt (or low-fat mayonnaise)

- 4 tbsp. low fat harsh cream

- 2 tsps. nectar

- 1 cup destroyed carrots

- 1/2 cup green onions, minced

- 1 tbsp. lemon juice

- 1 tsp. paprika

- 1/2 tsp. garlic powder

- 1/2 tsp. onion powder

- 1/2 tsp. dark pepper

- 1/2 tsp. oregano

- 1/2 tsp. cumin

- 1/8 tsp. cayenne pepper (or more)

- Salt to taste

Direction:

1. Combine the yogurt, harsh cream, lemon, nectar, and all the flavors.

2. Include the chicken, carrots, and green onions.

3. Taste and season with salt, pepper, or cayenne.

Nutrition:

- **Calories:** 173 Cal

- **Fat:** 21 g

- **Carbs:** 5 g

- **Protein:** 6 g

- **Fiber:** 2 g

Vinaigrette with Blue Cheese

Preparation Time: 5 Minutes

Cooking Time: 5 Minutes

Servings: 2

Ingredients:

- 2 hearts romaine, hacked

- 1 clove garlic, hacked

- 1/2 teaspoon dried oregano leaves

- 2 teaspoons sugar

- 2 tablespoons red wine vinegar

- 1/4 cup extra-virgin olive oil

- 1/4 pound blue cheddar disintegrates, in claim to fame cheddar segment of your market

- Salt and pepper

Direction:

1. Spot lettuce in a major bowl. Consolidate garlic, oregano, sugar and vinegar in a little bowl.

2. Add oil to dressing in a moderate stream and blend in with a whisk or fork and mix in blue cheddar.

3. Pour dressing over plate of mixed greens and hurl.

4. Season with salt and pepper, to taste.

Nutrition:

- **Calories:** 128 Cal

- **Fat:** 16 g

- **Carbs:** 2 g

- **Protein:** 5 g

- **Fiber:** 2.1 g

Mint Raita grilled Chicken with Tandoori

Preparation Time: 20 Minutes

Cooking Time: 45 Minutes

Servings: 4

Ingredients:

- 2 tablespoons hacked stripped new ginger

- 1 tablespoon paprika

- 1 tablespoon new lime juice

- 1 teaspoon stew powder

- 3/4 teaspoon salt

- 1/2 teaspoon ground turmeric

- 1/2 teaspoon ground cumin

- 1/8 teaspoon ground red pepper

- 3 garlic cloves, cleaved

- 4 (12-ounce) bone-in chicken leg-thigh quarters, cleaned Raita:

- 3/4 cup sans fat Greek yogurt

- 3/4 cup slashed seeded cucumber

- 2 tablespoons cleaved crisp mint

21

- 1/2 teaspoon ground cumin

- 1/4 teaspoon salt Cooking shower

Direction:

1. To set up the marinade, join initial 10 fixings in a blender; process until smooth. Fill an enormous zip-top plastic sack. Include chicken; go to cover. Marinate chicken in cooler for at any rate 4 hours or medium-term.

2. To set up the raita, join 3/4 cup yogurt and remaining fixings aside from cooking shower in a little bowl; cover and refrigerate.

3. Expel chicken from the cooler, and let remain at room temperature for 45 minutes.

4. Set up the flame broil for aberrant barbecuing. On the off chance that utilizing a gas flame broil, heat one side to medium-high and leave one side with no warmth. On the off chance that utilizing a charcoal barbecue, orchestrate hot coals on either side of the charcoal mesh, leaving an unfilled space in the center.

5. Expel the chicken from marinade, and dispose of the rest of the marinade. Spot the chicken on an unheated piece of flame broil rack covered with cooking shower. Close top, and barbecue for an hour and a half or until a thermometer embedded into a substantial piece of the thigh register 165°, turning chicken like clockwork.

Nutrition:

- **Calories:** 298 Cal

- **Fat:** 20 g

- **Carbs:** 4 g

- **Protein:** 8 g

- **Fiber:** 3 g

Salmon Salad with Feta Cheese

Preparation Time: 10 Minutes

Cooking Time: 10 Minutes

Servings: 2

Ingredients:

- 10 ounces' salmon fillet, wild-caught

- 8 cherry tomatoes, diced

- ½ head of Romaine lettuce, cut into bite-sized pieces

- 1-ounce Kalamata olives

- 4 ounces' cucumber, diced

- 2 tablespoons mint, chopped

- ¼ of a medium red onion, peeled and sliced

- 1/3 teaspoon salt

- ¼ teaspoon ground black pepper

- 1 tablespoon lemon juice

- 1 tablespoon avocado oil

- 4 ounces' feta cheese, full-fat, crumbled

Dressing

- ½ of lemon, juiced

- 1 medium avocado, peeled and pitted

- ¼ teaspoon salt

- ¼ teaspoon ground black pepper

- ½ teaspoon minced garlic

- 2 tablespoons avocado oil

Direction:

1. Take a griddle pan, place it over medium-high heat, add oil, and let it heat.

2. Season salmon with salt and black pepper, place it on the heated pan, and cook for 4–5 minutes per side until seared.

3. Meanwhile, take a large salad bowl, place in it the remaining ingredients for the salad, and toss until mixed.

4. Prepare the dressing and for this, place all of its ingredients in a blender and pulse until smooth.

5. When salmon has cooked, transfer it to a cutting board, cool for 5 minutes, and cut it into slices.

6. Arrange salmon slices over the salad, drizzle with the salad dressing, and then serve.

Nutrition:

- **Calories:** 138 Cal

- **Fat:** 21 g

- **Carbs:** 5 g

- **Protein:** 9 g

- **Fiber:** 2 g

Spicy Shrimp Salad

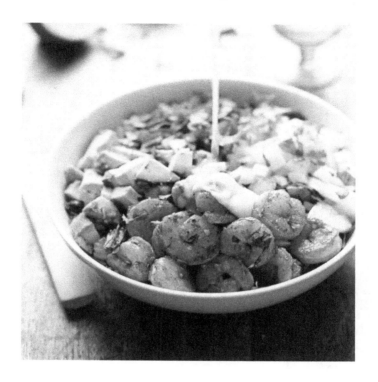

Preparation Time: 10 Minutes

Cooking Time: 8 Minutes

Servings: 2

Ingredients:

- 10 ounces' shrimps, peeled and deveined

- 2 medium avocados; peeled, pitted, diced

- ½ teaspoon minced garlic

- 5 ounces' cucumber, peeled and sliced

- ½ of a lime, juiced

- 2 ounces' baby spinach

- 2/3 teaspoon salt

- 2 teaspoons red chili powder

- ¼ teaspoon ground black pepper

- 3 tablespoons avocado oil

Dressing

- ½ teaspoon minced garlic

- 1 tablespoon ginger, grated

- ¼ teaspoon salt

- ¼ teaspoon ground black pepper

- ½ of a lime, juiced

- ½ tablespoon soy sauce

- ¼ cup avocado oil

Direction:

1. Take a medium-sized bowl, place avocado slices in it, and drizzle with one-fourth of the lime juice.

2. Take a shallow dish or a plate, place avocado slices in it, add cucumber and spinach, sprinkle with 1/3 teaspoon salt, and toss until combined.

3. Take a large frying pan, place it over medium heat, add oil, and when hot, add garlic and red chili powder and cook for 1 minute until beginning to turn golden-brown.

4. Add shrimps, cook for 2–3 minutes until pink, flip the shrimps, and continue cooking for another 2–3 minutes until cooked.

5. When done, transfer shrimps to a plate, season with remaining salt and black pepper, and arrange them on top of the vegetables.

6. Prepare the dressing, and for this, place all of its ingredients in the blender, pulse until well combined, and then drizzle over the salad.

7. Serve straight away.

Nutrition:

- **Calories:** 201 Cal

- **Fat:** 21 g

- **Carbs:** 5 g

- **Protein:** 5 g

- **Fiber:** 2 g

Keto Mustard Salad

Preparation Time: 15 Minutes

Cooking Time: 0 Minutes

Servings: 2

Ingredients:

- ½ pound green cabbage, cored and shredded

- ½ of a lemon, juiced

- 1 tablespoon Dijon mustard

- 1/8 teaspoon fennel seeds

- 1 teaspoon salt

- 1/8 teaspoon ground black pepper

- ½ cup mayonnaise, full-fat

Direction:

1. Take a medium-sized bowl, place shredded cabbage in it, sprinkle with salt, and drizzle with lemon juice.

2. Toss until combined and then let the cabbage rest for 10 minutes until slightly wilted.

3. Drain the cabbage, add mustard, salt, black pepper, fennel seeds, and mayonnaise, and stir until well mixed.

Nutrition:

- **Calories:** 209 Cal

- **Fat:** 21 g

- **Carbs**: 4 g

- **Protein:** 8 g

- **Fiber:** 3 g

Warm Kale Salad

Preparation Time: 10 Minutes

Cooking Time: 5 Minutes

Servings: 4

Ingredients:

- 8 ounces' kale, destemmed and cut into small pieces

- ½ teaspoon minced garlic

- 1/3 teaspoon salt

- ¼ teaspoon ground black pepper

- 1 teaspoon Dijon mustard

- 2 tablespoons avocado oil

- 2 tablespoons mayonnaise, full-fat

- 2 ounces unsalted butter

- ¾ cup heavy whipping cream, full-fat

- 4 ounces' feta cheese, full-fat

Direction:

1. Prepare the dressing and for this, take a medium-sized bowl, pour in oil, cream, mayonnaise; add mustard, garlic, salt, and black pepper. Whisk until well combined and set aside until needed.

2. Take a large frying pan, place it over medium heat, add butter, and when it melts, add kale leaves.

3. Toss until coated, cook for 3 minutes, and season with salt and black pepper.

4. Transfer kale to the bowl, pour the prepared dressing over the kale, and stir until mixed.

5. Top feta cheese over kale and then serve.

Nutrition:

- **Calories:** 488 Cal

- **Fat:** 27 g

- **Carbs:** 4 g

- **Protein:** 8 g

- **Fiber:** 3 g

Broccoli Salad with Dill

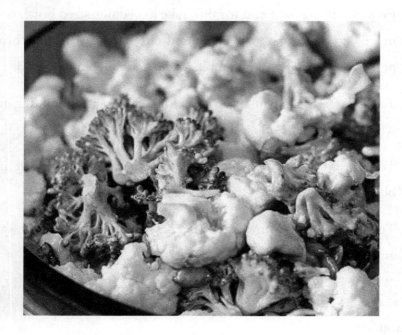

Preparation Time: 15 Minutes

Cooking Time: 10 Minutes

Servings: 4

Ingredients:

- 1 pound head of broccoli

- 4 slices of bacon, cooked and crumbled

- 1/3 teaspoon salt

- ¾ cup dill, fresh

- ¼ teaspoon ground black pepper

- 1 cup mayonnaise, full-fat

Direction:

1. Prepare the broccoli and for this, cut its florets and stem into very small pieces.

2. Take a large pot half full with salty water, place it over medium-high heat, and bring it to a boil.

3. Add broccoli florets and stems into the boiling water, boil for 5 minutes (or more, until fork-tender but crisp), and drain.

4. Place broccoli florets and stem into a large bowl and let it cool for 10 minutes.

5. Add remaining ingredients and stir until mixed.

6. Serve straight away.

Nutrition:

- **Calories:** 418 Cal

- **Fat:** 12 g

- **Carbs:** 5 g

- **Protein:** 9g

- **Fiber:** 3 g

Collagen Mug Cake

Preparation Time: 5 Minutes

Cooking Time: 2 Minutes

Servings: 1

Ingredients:

- 2 eggs, pasteurized, at room temperature

- 1 scoop of keto collagen

- ¼ teaspoon of sea salt

- ½ teaspoon baking powder

- 1 tablespoon cacao powder, unsweetened

- 10 drops of liquid stevia

- 1 tablespoon sunflower butter

- 1 teaspoon clarified butter

- 2 tablespoons coconut milk, full-fat

Direction:

1. Take a large microwave-proof mug, crack eggs in it, add sunflower butter and milk, and whisk until blended.

2. Add cacao powder, salt, and baking powder, stir until combined, and whisk in collagen until smooth.

3. Place the mug into the microwave and cook for 2 minutes on high heat until done.

4. When done, drizzle clarified butter over the cake and then serve.

Nutrition:

- **Calories:** 418 Cal

- **Fat:** 10 g

- **Carbs:** 4 g

- **Protein:** 27 g

- **Fiber:** 3 g

Chocolate and Nut Butter Cups

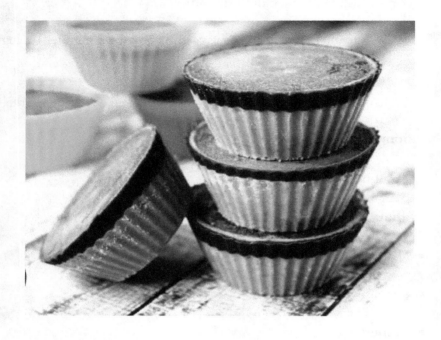

Preparation Time: 35 Minutes

Cooking Time: 2 Minutes

Servings: 6

Ingredients:

- 1-ounce chocolate, unsweetened

- 1/3 cup stevia

- 1 stick of unsalted butter

- 4 tablespoons peanut butter

- 2 tablespoons heavy cream

Direction:

1. Take a medium-sized bowl, place unsalted butter in it, and then microwave for 1–2 minutes until butter melts, stirring every 30 seconds.

2. Add stevia, peanut butter, and cream, and then stir until combined.

3. Take a muffin tray, line six cups with a cupcake liner, fill them evenly with chocolate mixture, and freeze for a minimum of 30 minutes until firm.

4. Serve straight away.

Nutrition:

- **Calories:** 120 Cal

- **Fat:** 17 g

- **Carbs:** 5 g

- **Protein:** 9 g

- **Fiber:** 12 g

Peanut Butter Cup Chaffle

Preparation Time: 10 Minutes

Cooking Time: 20 Minutes

Servings: 4

Ingredients:

Chaffle:

- 2 teaspoons coconut flour

- 2 tablespoons cocoa powder, unsweetened

- ½ teaspoon baking powder

- 2 tablespoons swerve sweetener

- 1 teaspoon vanilla extract, unsweetened

- 1 teaspoon cake batter extract, unsweetened

- 4 tablespoons heavy cream, full-fat

- 4 eggs, pasteurized, at room temperature

Filling:

- 4 teaspoons erythritol sweetener

- 6 tablespoons peanut butter

- 4 tablespoons heavy cream, full-fat

40

Direction:

1. Switch on the waffle maker and set it to preheat according to the manufacturer's instructions.

2. Meanwhile, prepare the batter and for this, take a medium-sized bowl, add all the ingredients to it, and whisk well by using an electric mixer at medium speed until incorporated and smooth batter comes together.

3. Grease the waffle maker with avocado oil spray and ladle the prepared batter on waffle trays.

4. Shut the waffle maker with its lid and let cook for 5–8 minutes until waffle turns firm and golden-brown.

5. When done, remove waffles by using a tong or a fork and repeat with the remaining batter.

6. While chaffle cooks, prepare the filling, and for this, take a medium-sized bowl, place all of its ingredients in it, and whisk until combined.

7. Let waffles cool slightly, spread the prepared filling on top, sandwich two chaffles together, and serve.

Nutrition:

- **Calories:** 128 Cal

- **Fat:** 17 g

- **Carbs:** 4 g

- **Protein:** 9g

- **Fiber:** 3 g

Cinnamon Sugar Chaffle

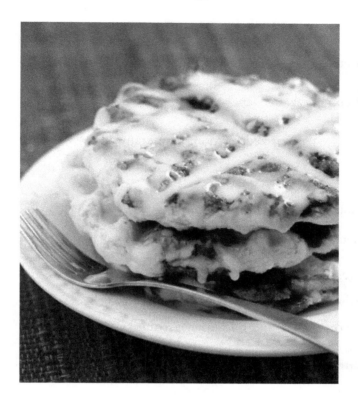

Preparation Time: 10 Minutes

Cooking Time: 20 Minutes

Servings: 4

Ingredients:

- 8 tablespoons almond flour

- 2 teaspoons ground cinnamon

- 8 tablespoons erythritol sweeteners

43

- 1 teaspoon baking powder

- 4 teaspoons vanilla extract, unsweetened

- 4 tablespoons sour cream, full-fat

- 1 cup mozzarella cheese, full-fat, shredded

- 4 eggs, pasteurized, at room temperature

Direction:

1. Switch on the waffle maker and set it to preheat according to the manufacturer's instructions.

2. Meanwhile, prepare the batter and for this, take a medium-sized bowl, add all the ingredients (except for cheese), whisk well until incorporated, and fold in cheese until combined.

3. Grease the waffle maker with avocado oil spray and ladle the prepared batter on waffle trays.

4. Shut the waffle maker with its lid and let cook for 5–8 minutes until waffle turns firm and golden-brown.

5. When done, remove waffles by using a tong or a fork and repeat with the remaining batter.

6. Let waffles cool slightly and serve

Nutrition:

- **Calories:** 267 Cal

- **Fat:** 10 g

- **Carbs:** 4 g

- **Protein:** 8 g

- **Fiber:** 3 g

<u>Cinnamon and Cream Cheese Chaffle</u>

Preparation Time: 10 Minutes

Cooking Time: 20 Minutes

Servings: 4

Ingredients:

- 4 tablespoons almond flour

- 2 tablespoons erythritol sweetener

- 2 teaspoons ground cinnamon

- 1 teaspoon baking powder

- 2 tablespoons whey protein powder, unflavored

- ½ teaspoon vanilla extract, unsweetened

- 2 eggs, pasteurized, at room temperature

- ½ cup cream cheese, full-fat, softened

Direction:

1. Switch on the waffle maker and set it to preheat according to the manufacturer's instructions.

2. Meanwhile, prepare the batter and for this, take a medium-sized bowl, crack eggs in it, add cinnamon and sweetener, and whisk well by using an electric mixer at medium speed until fluffy.

46

3. Add remaining ingredients and whisk until incorporated and smooth batter comes together.

4. Grease the waffle maker with avocado oil spray and ladle the prepared batter on waffle trays.

5. Shut the waffle maker with its lid and let cook for 5–8 minutes until waffle turns firm and golden-brown.

6. When done, remove waffles by using a tong or a fork and repeat with the remaining batter.

7. Let waffles cool slightly and serve.

Nutrition:

- **Calories:** 225 Cal

- **Fat:** 22 g

- **Carbs:** 6 g

- **Protein:** 4 g

- **Fiber:** 8 g

Golden Chaffles

Preparation Time: 10 Minutes

Cooking Time: 20 Minutes

Servings: 4

Ingredients:

- 6 tablespoons almond flour

- 1 ½ teaspoon baking powder

- 1 tablespoon erythritol sweetener

- 1 teaspoon vanilla extract, unsweetened

- 4 eggs, pasteurized, at room temperature

- 2 1/3 cups mozzarella cheese, full-fat, shredded

Direction:

1. Switch on the waffle maker and set it to preheat according to the manufacturer's instructions.

2. Meanwhile, prepare the batter and for this, take a medium-sized bowl, place flour in it, add baking powder and sweetener, and stir until combined.

3. Then add vanilla, cheese, and eggs, and whisk well by using an electric mixer at medium speed until incorporated and smooth batter comes together.

4. Grease the waffle maker with avocado oil spray and ladle the prepared batter on waffle trays.

5. Shut the waffle maker with its lid and then let cook for 5–8 minutes until the waffle turns firm and golden-brown.

6. When done, remove waffles by using a tong or a fork and repeat with the remaining batter.

7. Let waffles cool slightly and serve.

Nutrition:

*   **Calories:** 168 Cal

*   **Fat:** 10 g

*   **Carbs:** 2 g

*   **Protein:** 4 g

*   **Fiber:** 3 g

Churro Chaffle

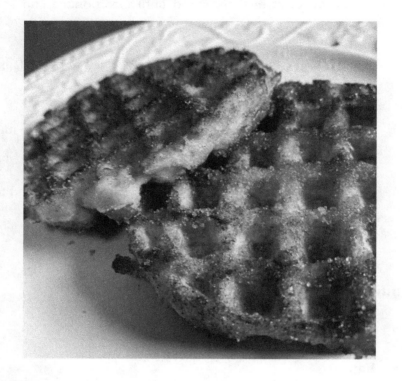

Preparation Time: 10 Minutes

Cooking Time: 20 Minutes

Servings: 4

Ingredients:

Chaffle:

- 8 teaspoons coconut flour

- 4 teaspoons pumpkin pie spice

- 8 tablespoons swerve sweetener

- 1 teaspoon baking powder

- 2 teaspoons vanilla extract, unsweetened

- 4 eggs, pasteurized, at room temperature

- 4 tablespoons unsalted butter, melted

- 2 cups mozzarella cheese, full-fat, shredded

Topping:

- 2 2/3 teaspoons ground cinnamon

- 1 cup swerve sweetener

- 1 1/3 teaspoons ground nutmeg

- 8 tablespoons unsalted butter, melted

Direction:

1. Switch on the waffle maker and set it to preheat according to the manufacturer's instructions.

2. Meanwhile, prepare the batter and for this, take a medium-sized bowl, add all the ingredients to it, and whisk well by using an electric mixer at medium speed until incorporated and smooth batter comes together.

3. Grease the waffle maker with avocado oil spray and ladle the prepared batter on waffle trays.

4. Shut the waffle maker with its lid and let cook for 5–8 minutes until waffle turns firm and golden-brown.

5. When done, remove waffles by using a tong or a fork and repeat with the remaining batter.

6. While Chaffle cooks, prepare the topping, and for this, take a medium-sized bowl, place cinnamon, sweetener, and nutmeg, and stir until mixed.

7. Let waffles cool slightly, brush with butter, sprinkle cinnamon mixture on top, and serve.

Nutrition:

- **Calories:** 212 Cal

- **Fat:** 19 g

- **Carbs:** 5 g

- **Protein:** 4 g

- **Fiber:** 2 g

Yogurt Chaffle

Preparation Time: 10 Minutes

Cooking Time: 20 Minutes

Servings: 4

Ingredients:

- 2 cups mozzarella cheese, full-fat, shredded

- 4 eggs, pasteurized, at room temperature

- 8 tablespoons ground almonds

- 2 teaspoons psyllium husk

- 2 teaspoons baking powder

- 4 tablespoons yogurt, full-fat

Direction:

1. Switch on the waffle maker and set it to preheat according to the manufacturer's instructions.

2. Meanwhile, prepare the batter and for this, take a medium-sized bowl, add all the ingredients, whisk well by using an electric mixer at medium speed until incorporated, and let the mixture sit for 5 minutes.

3. Grease the waffle maker with avocado oil spray and ladle the prepared batter on waffle trays.

4. Shut the waffle maker with its lid and let cook for 5–8 minutes until waffle turns firm and golden-brown.

5. When done, remove waffles by using a tong or a fork and repeat with the remaining batter.

6. Let waffles cool slightly and serve.

Nutrition:

- **Calories:** 131 Cal

- **Fat:** 6 g

- **Carbs:** 3 g

- **Protein:** 9 g

- **Fiber:** 3 g

Zucchini Chaffle

Preparation Time: 10 Minutes

Cooking Time: 20 Minutes

Servings: 4

Ingredients:

- 2 cups zucchini, grated

- 1 ½ teaspoon salt, divided

- 1 teaspoon ground black pepper

- 2 teaspoons dried basil

- 1 cup parmesan cheese, full-fat, shredded

- 2 eggs, pasteurized, at room temperature

- ½ cup mozzarella cheese, shredded

Direction:

1. Place grated zucchini in a colander, sprinkle with ¼ teaspoon salt, toss until mixed, and then let it sit for 5 minutes.

2. Meanwhile, switch on the waffle maker and set it to preheat according to the manufacturer's instructions.

3. After 5 minutes, wrap grated zucchini in a paper towel and press tightly to squeeze out moisture as much as possible.

4. Meanwhile, prepare the batter and for this, take a medium-sized bowl, crack the eggs in it, and whisk until blended.

5. Add zucchini in it along with remaining salt, black pepper, basil, and mozzarella cheese, and stir until mixed.

6. Grease the waffle maker with avocado oil spray, sprinkle 2 tablespoons of parmesan cheese on waffle trays until covered, and ladle the prepared batter on top.

7. Top batter with another 2 tablespoons of parmesan cheese, shut the waffle maker with its lid, and let cook for 5–8 minutes until waffle turns firm and golden-brown.

8. When done, remove waffles by using a tong or a fork and repeat with the remaining batter and parmesan cheese.

9. Let waffles cool slightly and serve

Nutrition:

- **Calories:** 128 Cal

- **Fat:** 9 g

- **Carbs:** 7 g

- **Protein:** 8 g

- **Fiber:** 5 g

Cauliflower Chaffle

Preparation Time: 10 Minutes

Cooking Time: 20 Minutes

Servings: 4

Ingredients:

- 2 cups cauliflower florets, grated

- ½ teaspoon garlic powder

- ½ teaspoon salt

- ½ teaspoon ground black pepper

- 1 teaspoon Italian seasoning

- 2 eggs, pasteurized, at room temperature

- 1 cup mozzarella cheese, full-fat, shredded

- 1 cup parmesan cheese, full-fat, shredded

Direction:

1. Switch on the waffle maker and set it to preheat according to the manufacturer's instructions.

2. Meanwhile, prepare the batter and for this, take a medium-sized bowl, add all the ingredients to it, and whisk well by using an

electric mixer at medium speed until incorporated and smooth batter comes together.

3. Grease the waffle maker with avocado oil spray, sprinkle 2 tablespoons of parmesan cheese on waffle trays until covered, and ladle the prepared batter on top.

4. Shut the waffle maker with its lid and let cook for 5–8 minutes until waffle turns firm and golden-brown.

5. When done, remove waffles by using a tong or a fork and repeat with the remaining batter.

6. Let waffles cool slightly and serve.

Nutrition:

- **Calories:** 290 Cal

- **Fat:** 13 g

- **Carbs:** 5 g

- **Protein:** 9 g

- **Fiber:** 4 g

Zesty Chili Lime Tuna Salad

Preparation Time: 10 Minutes

Cooking Time: 0 Minutes

Servings: 4

Ingredients:

- 1 tablespoon of lime juice

- 1/3 cup of mayonnaise

- ¼ teaspoon of salt

- 1 teaspoon of Tajin chili lime seasoning

- 1/8 teaspoon of pepper

- 1 medium stalk celery (finely chopped)

- 2 cups of romaine lettuce (chopped roughly)

- 2 tablespoons of red onion (finely chopped)

- optional: chopped green onion, black pepper, lemon juice

- 5 ozs. canned tuna

Direction:

1. Using a bowl of medium size, mix some of the ingredients such as lime, pepper and chili lime

2. Then, add tuna and vegetables to the pot and stir. You can serve with cucumber, celery or a bed of greens

Nutrition:

- **Calories:**409 Cal

- **Fat:** 37 g

- **Carbs:** 4 g

- **Protein:** 9 g

- **Fiber:** 3 g

Sheet Pan Brussels Sprouts and Bacon

Preparation Time: 5 Minutes

Cooking Time: 35 Minutes

Servings: 4

Ingredients:

- 6 ozs. bacon

- 6 ozs. raw brussels sprouts

- Salt

- Pepper

Direction:

- Prepare the oven by preheating it to 400 degrees, Then, prepare the baking sheet with parchment paper

- Prepare brussels sprouts in the pan

- Use kitchen shears to cut the bacon into little pieces

- Add the cut bacon and brussels sprouts into the baking sheet already prepared. Then, add pepper and salt

- Bake for up to 45 minutes. Allow the Brussel sprouts to become crispy

Nutrition:

- **Calories:** 138 Cal

- **Fat:** 20 g

- **Carbs:** 6 g

- **Protein:** 7 g

- **Fiber:** 4 g

Super Simple Chicken Cauliflower Fried Rice

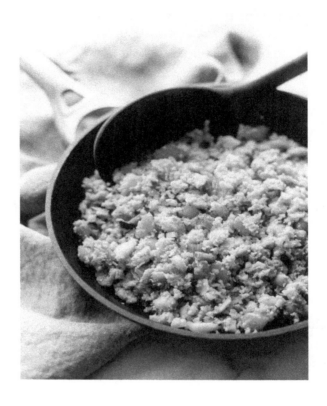

Preparation Time: 5 Minutes

Cooking Time: 20 Minutes

Servings: 4

Ingredients:

- ½ teaspoon of sesame oil

- 1 small carrot (chopped)

- 1 tablespoon of avocado or coconut oil

- 1 small onion (finely sliced)

- ½ cup of snap peas (chopped)

- ½ cup of red peppers cut finely

- 1 tablespoon of garlic

- 1 tablespoon of garlic, properly chopped

- 1 teaspoon of salt

- 2 teaspoons of garlic powder

- 4 chicken breasts, chopped and cooked

- 4 cups of rice cauliflower

- 2 large scrambled eggs

- Gluten-free soy sauce, one quarter cup size

Direction:

1. Gently season the chicken breasts with ½ tablespoon of salt, ¼ tablespoon of pepper, and ½ tablespoon of olive oil. Cook the chicken on any pan of your choice

2. Add coconut/olive/avocado oil. Cut some onions and carrots and sauce and leave for up to 3 minutes

3. Next, add the rest of the vegetables, pepper/salt/garlic powder and then cook for extra 3 minutes

4. Put in fresh garlic coconut aminos or soy sauce and riced cauliflower; then stir

5. Add scrambled eggs and chicken and mix until they are well combined

6. Put off the heat and then stir in some green peas. Season again, you can top it with sesame seeds if you like

Nutrition:

- **Calories:** 260 Cal

- **Fat:** 21 g

- Carbs: 6 g

- **Protein:** 3 g

- **Fiber:** 4 g

Prep-Ahead Low-Carb Casserole

Preparation Time: 5 Minutes

Cooking Time: 35 Minutes

Servings: 4

Ingredients:

- 1 cooked and cubed chicken breast

- 4 cooked and crumbled strips of bacon

- ½ cup of celery, chopped

- 1/3 cup of mozzarella cheese

- 1 tablespoon of Italian seasoning

- ½ cup of grated parmesan

- 3 whisked eggs

- ¼ whipping cream

Direction:

1. Start by pre-heating the oven to at least above 350 degrees °F. Use a non-stick cooking spray to spray a casserole dish

2. Combine all the ingredients, leaving out the only mozzarella with a mixing bowl. Continue mixing until properly combined

3. Pour out the mixture into a casserole dish. You can top it with mozzarella

4. Bake for up to 35 minutes. Then, increase the heat and allow to boil until the mozzarella turns to golden brown

5. Allow it to cool before serving

Nutrition:

- **Calories:** 234 Cal

- **Fat:** 20 g

- **Carbs:** 3 g

- **Protein:** 9 g

- **Fiber:** 2 g

BBQ Pulled Beef Sando

Preparation Time: 5 Minutes

Cooking Time: 10-12 Hours

Servings: 4

Ingredients:

- 3 lbs. boneless chuck roasts

- 2 tablespoons of pink Himalayan salt

- 2 tablespoons of garlic powder

- 1 tablespoon of onion powder

- ¼ apple cider vinegar

- 2 tablespoons of coconut aminos

- ½ cup of bone broth

- ¼ cup of melted Kerry gold butter

- 1 tablespoon of black pepper

- 1 tablespoon of smoked paprika

- 2 tablespoons of tomato paste

Direction:

1. Trim the fat from the beef and slice it into two huge pieces

2. Mix salt, onion, paprika, black pepper, and garlic. Next is to rub the mixture on the beef and then put the beef in a slow cooker

3. Use another bowl to melt butter. Then, add a tomato paste, coconut aminos, and vinegar. Pour it all over the beef. Next is to add the bone broth into the slow cooker by pouring it around the beef

4. Cook for about 10 minutes. After that, take out the beef and increase the temperature of the cooker so that the sauce can thicken. Tear the beef before adding it to the slow cooker and toss with the sauce

Nutrition:

- **Calories:** 184 Cal

- **Fat:** 29 g

- **Carbs:** 7 g

- **Protein:** 11 g

- **Fiber:** 2 g

Keto-friendly Oatmeal Recipe

Preparation Time: 5 Minutes

Cooking Time: 15 Minutes

Servings: 4

Ingredients:

- 1 tablespoon of flaxseed meal

- ½ cup of hemp hearts

- 1 tablespoon of chia seeds

- 1 tablespoon coconut flakes

- 1 cup of unsweetened almond milk

- 1 scoop of Vanilla MCT oil powder (1 tablespoon of coconut oil and 1 tablespoon of stevia)

- 1 teaspoon of cinnamon

Direction:

1. Add all the ingredients in a saucepot and mix

2. Stir until it simmers and is thick enough to your liking

3. You can serve garnished with frozen berries

Nutrition:

- **Calories:** 189 Cal

- **Fat:** 22 g

- **Carbs:** 4 g

- **Protein:** 9 g

- **Fiber:** 5 g

Crunchy Coconut Cluster Keto Cereal

Preparation Time: 5 Minutes

Cooking Time: 20 Minutes

Servings: 4

Ingredients:

- ½ cup of unsweetened shredded coconut

- ½ cup of hemp hearts

- ½ cup of raw pumpkin seeds

- A pinch of sea salt

- 2 scoops of perfect Keto MCT oil powder

- 1 white egg

- 1 teaspoon of cinnamon

Direction:

1. The oven should be pre-heated to 350° F

2. A sheet pan should then be lined with parchment paper

3. Stir all the dry ingredients in the bowl

4. Using a separate bowl, mix the white egg until it becomes frothy. Then, pour it slowly into the dry; mix

5. Transfer the mixture into a sheet of the pan and flatten to a thickness of ¼ of an inch

6. Leave to bake for 15 minutes. After removal, use a spatula to break up the mass into chunks and allow to bake for more 5 minutes

7. Finally, take it out of the oven and serve with your milk of choice. It can be stored for three days in an airtight container at room temperature

Nutrition:

- **Calories:** 5258 Cal

- **Fat:** 25 g

- **Carbs:** 7 g

- **Protein:** 9 g

- **Fiber:** 2 g

Avocado Egg Bowls

Preparation Time: 5 Minutes

Cooking Time: 15 Minutes

Servings: 4

Ingredients:

- 1 avocado halved with the removed stone

- 1 tablespoon of salted butter

- 3 free-range eggs

- 3 rashers of bacon into little pieces

- Black pepper and pinch of salt

Direction:

1. Begin by removing most of the avocado flesh, remaining just ½ inch on the avocado

2. Put in butter into a large saucepan while it's heating. Let the butter melt in the pan. Crack the eggs and beat them in a jug, adding a little pepper and salt

3. Put the bacon on one side of the pan and leave everything to fry for some minutes. Next, add the eggs to the opposite bottom of the pan and continue to stir until it is scrambled. The bacon and the eggs should be ready soon enough in 5 minutes. In case the

74

scrambled eggs are done before the bacon, take it from the pan into a bowl

4. Mix the pieces of the bacon and the scrambled eggs in the pot and add into the avocado bowls

Nutrition:

- **Calories:** 500 Cal

- **Fat:** 26 g

- **Carbs:** 6 g

- **Protein:** 9 g

- **Fiber:** 9 g

Keto Cinnamon Coffee

Preparation Time: 5 Minutes

Cooking Time: 5 Minutes

Servings: 1

Ingredients:

- 2 tbsps. ground coffee

- 1/3 cup of heavy whipping cream

- 1 tsp. ground cinnamon

- 2 cups water

Direction:

1. Start by mixing the cinnamon with the ground coffee.

2. Pour in hot water and do what you usually do when brewing. Use a mixer or whisk to whip the cream 'til you get stiff peaks Serve in a tall mug and put the whipped cream on the surface. Sprinkle with some cinnamon and enjoy.

Nutrition:

- **Calories:** 168 Cal

- **Fat:** 18 g

- **Carbs:** 7 g

- **Protein:** 9 g

- **Fiber:** 3 g

Keto Waffles and Blueberries

Preparation Time: 5 Minutes

Cooking Time: 15 Minutes

Servings: 8

Ingredients:

- 8 eggs

- 5 ozs. melted butter

- 1 tsp. vanilla extract

- 2 tsps. baking powder

- 1/3 cup coconut flour

- 3 ozs. butter (topping)

- 1 oz. fresh blueberries (topping)

Direction:

1. Start by mixing the butter and eggs first until you get a smooth batter. Put in the remaining ingredients except those that we'll be using as topping.

2. Heat your waffle iron to medium temperature and start pouring in the batter for cooking

3. In a separate bowl, mix the butter and blueberries using a hand mixer. Use this to top off your freshly cooked waffles

Nutrition:

- **Calories:** 504 Cal

- **Fat:** 21 g

- **Carbs:** 5 g

- **Protein:** 7 g

- **Fiber:** 4 g

Baked Avocado Eggs

Preparation Time: 5 Minutes

Cooking Time: 30 Minutes

Servings: 4

Ingredients:

- Avocados

- 4 eggs

- ½ cup of bacon bits, around 55 grams

- 2 tbsps. fresh chives, chopped

- 1 sprig of chopped fresh basil, chopped

- 1 cherry tomato, quartered

- Salt and pepper to taste

- Shredded cheddar cheese

Direction:

1. Start by preheating the oven to 400 degrees Fahrenheit

2. Slice the avocado and remove the pits. Put them on a baking sheet and crack some eggs onto the center hole of the avocado. If it's too small, just scoop out more of the flesh to make room. Salt and pepper to taste.

3. Top with bacon bits and bake for 15 minutes. Remove and sprinkle with herbs. Enjoy!

Nutrition:

- **Calories:** 271 Cal

- **Fat:** 18 g

- **Carbs:** 7 g

- **Protein:** 9 g

- **Fiber:** 3 g

Mushroom Omelet

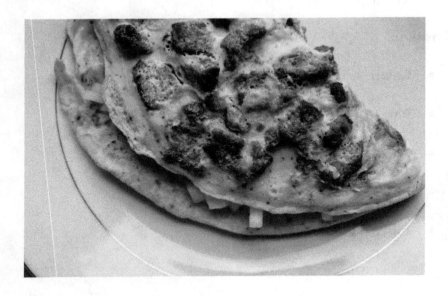

Preparation Time: 5 Minutes

Cooking Time: 5 Minutes

Servings: 1

Ingredients:

- 3 eggs, medium

- 1 oz. shredded cheese

- 1 oz. butter used for frying

- ¼ yellow onion, chopped

- 4 large sliced mushrooms

- Your favorite vegetables, optional

- Salt and pepper to taste

Direction:

1. Crack and whisk the eggs in a bowl. Add some salt and pepper to taste.

2. Melt the butter in a pan using low heat. Put in the mushroom and onion, cooking the two until you get that amazing smell.

3. Pour the egg mix into the pan and allow it to cook on medium heat.

4. Allow the bottom part to cook before sprinkling the cheese on top of the still-raw portion of the egg.

5. Carefully pry the edges of the omelet and fold it in half. Allow it to cook for a few more seconds before removing the pan from the heat and sliding it directly onto your plate.

Nutrition:

- **Calories:** 528 Cal

- **Fat:** 25g

- **Carbs:** 8 g

- **Protein:** 11 g

- **Fiber:** 3 g

Chocolate Sea Salt Smoothie

Preparation Time: 5 Minutes

Cooking Time: 5 Minutes

Servings: 2

Ingredients:

- 1 avocado (frozen or not)

- 2 cups of almond milk

- 1 tbsp. tahini

- ¼ cup of cocoa powder

- 1 scoop Perfect Keto chocolate base

Direction:

Combine all the ingredients in a high-speed blender and mix until you get a soft smoothie.

Nutrition:

- **Calories:** 238 Cal
- **Fat:** 19 g
- **Carbs:** 3 g
- **Protein:** 14 g
- **Fiber:** 3 g

Zucchini Lasagna

Preparation Time: 20 Minutes

Cooking Time: 80 Minutes

Servings: 9

Ingredients:

- 3 cups raw macadamia nuts or soaked blanched almonds (for ricotta)

- 2 tbsps. nutritional yeast (for ricotta)

- 2 tsps. dried oregano (for ricotta)

- 1 tsp. sea salt (for ricotta)

- 1/2 cup water or more as needed (for ricotta)

- 1/4 cup vegan parmesan cheese (for ricotta)

- 1 cup fresh basil, chopped (for ricotta)

- 1 medium lemon, juiced (for ricotta)

- Black pepper to taste (for ricotta)

- 1 28-oz. jar favorite marinara sauce

- 3 medium zucchinis squash thinly sliced with a mandolin

Direction:

1. Preheat the oven to 375 degrees Fahrenheit Put macadamia nuts to a food processor.

2. Add the remaining ingredients and continue to puree the mixture. You want to create a fine paste.

3. Taste and adjust the seasonings depending on your personal preferences.

4. Pour 1 cup of marinara sauce in a baking dish.

5. Start creating the lasagna layers using thinly sliced zucchini

6. Scoop small amounts of ricotta mixture on the zucchini and spread it into a thin layer. Continue the layering until you've run out of zucchini or space for it.

7. Sprinkle parmesan cheese on the topmost layer.

8. Cover the pan with foil and bake for 45 minutes. Remove the foil and bake for 15 minutes more.

9. Allow it to cool for 15 minutes before serving. Serve immediately. The lasagna will keep for 3 days in the fridge.

Nutrition:

- **Calories:** 388 Cal

- **Fat:** 29 g

- **Carbs:** 9 g

- **Protein:** 10 g

- **Fiber:** 3 g

Vegan Keto Scramble

Preparation Time: 15 Minutes

Cooking Time: 10 Minutes

Servings: 2

Ingredients:

- 14 ozs. firm tofu

- 3 tbsps. avocado oil

- 2 tbsps. yellow onion, diced

- 1.5 tbsp. nutritional yeast

- ½ tsp. turmeric

- ½ tsp. garlic powder

- ½ tsp. salt

- 1 cup baby spinach

- 3 grape tomatoes

- 3 ozs. vegan cheddar cheese

Direction:

1. Start by squeezing the water out of the tofu block using a clean cloth or a paper towel.

2. Grab a skillet and put it on medium heat. Sauté the chopped onion in a small amount of avocado oil until it starts to caramelize

3. Using a potato masher, crumble the tofu on the skillet. Do this thoroughly until the tofu looks a lot like scrambled eggs.

4. Drizzle some more of the avocado oil onto the mix together with the dry seasonings. Stir thoroughly and evenly distribute the flavor.

5. Cook under medium heat, occasionally stirring to avoid burning of the tofu. You'd want most of the liquid to evaporate until you get a nice chunk of scrambled tofu. Fold the baby spinach, cheese, and diced tomato. Cook for a few more minutes until the cheese melted. Serve and enjoy!

Nutrition:

- **Calories:** 208 Cal

- **Fat:** 19 g

- **Carbs:** 9 g

- **Protein:** 10 g

- **Fiber:** 5 g

Parmesan Cheese Strips

Preparation Time: 20 Minutes

Cooking Time: 7 Minutes

Servings: 12

Ingredients:

1. 1 cup shredded parmesan cheese

2. 1 tsp dried basil

Direction:

1. Preheat the oven to 350 degrees Fahrenheit. Prepare the baking sheet by lining it with parchment paper.

2. Form small piles of the parmesan cheese on the baking sheet. Flatten it out evenly and then sprinkle dried basil on top of the cheese.

3. Bake for 5 to 7 minutes or until you get a golden-brown color with crispy edges. Take it out, serve, and enjoy!

Nutrition:

- **Calories:** 90 Cal

- **Fat:** 18 g

- **Carbs:** 7 g

- **Protein:** 9 g

- **Fiber:** 3 g

Peanut Butter Power Granola

Preparation Time: 5 Minutes

Cooking Time: 30 Minutes

Servings: 12

Ingredients:

- 1 cup shredded coconut or almond flour

- 1 1/2 cups almonds

- 1 1/2 cups pecans

- 1/3 cup swerve sweetener

- 1/3 cup vanilla whey protein, powder

- 1/3 cup peanut butter

- 1/4 cup sunflower seeds 1/4 cup butter

- 1/4 cup of water

Direction:

1. Preheat the oven to 300 degrees Fahrenheit and prepare a baking sheet with parchment paper

2. Place the almonds and pecans in a food processor. Put them all in a large bowl and add the sunflower seeds, shredded coconut, vanilla, sweetener, and protein powder.

93

3. Melt the peanut butter and butter together in the microwave. Mix the melted butter in the nut mixture and stir it thoroughly until the nuts are well-distributed.

4. Put in the water to create a lumpy mixture. Scoop out small amounts of the mixture and place it on the baking sheet.

5. Bake for 30 minutes. Enjoy!

Nutrition:

- **Calories:** 168 Cal

- **Fat:** 18 g

- **Carbs:** 7 g

- **Protein:** 9 g

- **Fiber:** 3 g

Homemade Graham Crackers

Preparation Time: 5 Minutes

Cooking Time: 30 Minutes

Servings: 10

Ingredients:

- 1 egg, large

- 2 cups almond flour

- 1/3 cup swerve brown

- 2 tsps. cinnamon

- 1 tsp. baking powder

- 2 tbsps. melted butter

- 1 tsp. vanilla extract

- Salt

Direction:

1. Preheat the oven to 300 degrees Fahrenheit

2. Grab a bowl and whisk the almond flour, cinnamon, sweetener, baking powder, and salt. Stir all the ingredients together.

3. Put in the egg, molasses, melted butter, and vanilla extract. Stir until you get a dough-like consistency.

4. Roll out the dough evenly, making sure that you don't go beyond ¼ of an inch thick. Cut the dough into the shapes you want for cooking. Transfer it on the baking tray

5. Bake for 20 to 30 minutes until it firms up. Let it cool for 30 minutes outside of the oven and then put them back in for another 30 minutes. Make sure that for the second time putting the biscuit, the temperature is not higher than 200 degrees Fahrenheit. This last step will make the biscuit crispy.

Nutrition:

- **Calories:** 158 Cal

- **Fat:** 21 g

- **Carbs:** 8 g

- **Protein:** 8 g

- **Fiber:** 3 g

Keto no-Bake Cookies

Preparation Time: 5 Minutes

Cooking Time: 10 Minutes

Servings: 18

Ingredients:

- 2/3 cup of all-natural peanut butter

- 1 cup of all-natural shredded coconut, unsweetened

- 2 tbsps. real butter

- 4 drops of vanilla

Direction:

1. Melt the butter in the microwave.

2. Take it out and put it in the peanut butter. Stir thoroughly. Add the sweetener and coconut. Mix.

3. Spoon it onto a pan lined with parchment paper Freeze for 10 minutes

4. Cut into preferred slices. Store in an airtight container in the fridge and enjoy whenever.

Nutrition:

- **Calories:** 80 Cal

- **Fat:** 21 g

- **Carbs:** 8 g

- **Protein:** 10 g

- **Fiber:** 3 g

Swiss Cheese Crunchy Nachos

Preparation Time: 5 Minutes

Cooking Time: 15 Minutes

Servings: 2

Ingredients:

- ½ cup shredded Swiss cheese

- ½ cup shredded cheddar cheese

- 1/8 cup cooked bacon pieces

Direction:

1. Preheat the oven to 300 degrees Fahrenheit and prepare the baking sheet by lining it with parchment paper.

2. Start by spreading the Swiss cheese on the parchment. Sprinkle it with bacon and then top it off again with the cheese.

3. Bake until the cheese has melted. This should take around 10 minutes or less.

4. Allow the cheese to cool before cutting them into triangle strips.

5. Grab another baking sheet and place the triangle cheese strips on top.

6. Broil them for 2 to 3 minutes so they'll get chunky.

Nutrition:

- **Calories:** 280 Cal

- **Fat:** 21 g

- **Carbs:** 5 g

- **Protein:** 9 g

- **Fiber:** 3 g

CONCLUSION

Thank you for reading all this book!

Tracking progress is something that straddles the fence. A lot of people say that this helps a lot of people and you can celebrate your wins, however, as everyone is different and they have different goals, progress can be slower in some than others. This can cause others to be frustrated and sad, as well as wanting to give up. One of the very most important things to remember is that while progress takes time, and you shouldn't get discouraged if you don't see results right away. With most diets, it takes at least a month to see any results. So, don't get discouraged and keep trying if your body is saying that you can. If you can't, then you will need to talk to your doctor and see if something else is for you.

You should make it a daily or everyday routine to try and lower your stress. Stress will not allow you to get into ketosis, which is that state that keto wants to put you in. The reason for this being that stress increases the hormone known as cortisol in your blood, and it will prevent your body from being able to burn fats for energy. This is because your body has too much sugar in your blood

You have already taken a step towards your improvement.

Best wishes!

CPSIA information can be obtained
at www.ICGtesting.com
Printed in the USA
BVHW061037220321
603178BV00004B/212

9 781802 223408